A Gentleman's Guide To

Choking The Chicken

How To Masturbate Like A Pro

G.R. Raleigh

Copyright Acknowledgment

Legal Disclaimer

Introduction

Choking one's chicken is something that, until now, has been something that men have had to learn on their own. This is not something that anyone ever teaches you. It's not shaving or how to ride a bike. Even when sex education comes up, masturbation is always left out. Additionally, alas, this is a subject that men, young and old alike, really hate discussing. We men often make fun of each other and use jerking off as an insult to our peers. There is never a frank discussion and there is certainly no comparing notes on what does and does work and what is and is not fun.

I started writing about sex and sexual topics, like this, some years back. I wanted to put my experiences out there, in a serious discussion and "how to" format. The topics that I have written about, are sadly the ones that are always left out of sex ed presentation, and even more sadly they are the ones that everyone seems to want to know about.

This is my latest attempt at bringing light into the darkness and instructing people how to have better, more enjoyable sex in a more confident manner. It is, as always, my sincere hope that you find this manual useful and helpful and that you experience a richer, more satisfying sex life because of it.

- G.R. Raleigh

Why Do Men Masturbate?

Well, simply put, masturbation is fun. There is nothing to be ashamed of. The same physical thrill of being with a partner can be experienced long before you ever get the chance. Really, it's just part of our lifestyle. First off, let me tell you that the vast majority of men masturbate. Those who are telling you that they don't are just part of the very, very tiny minority, or they are lying. Most likely lying. If you are thinking about, or are choking your chicken on a regular basis, you are **very** normal.

Let's face it. Men love sex. Men love having sex and thinking about sex. If there was the opportunity, I am sure that plenty of men would spend the day doing nothing but. It's not surprising. Our biology has programmed us to be keen on reproducing for one reason or another, so we are just that – keen on sex. However, there is a bit of a problem. We don't get to have sex all the time. Maybe we are too young and not ready for the emotional and social consequences of sex, maybe we are in between partners, maybe we're in a situation where sex isn't an option. Well, there is an option and that is self gratification.

Beyond just using masturbation as a way to have sex when sex is not an option, there are other reasons men masturbate. Like I said, it's fun. Cumming always feels good. Yes, it feels better with a partner but it still feels pretty damn good when you are alone. It's good for your mood as well. I find that when I get backed up, sexually speaking, I am just a bear to be around. I can't keep my mind straight and I find it hard to focus. Well, guess what? Whacking off clears all that up. Plenty of times I needed to jerk it before I finished a term paper, returned to my studies, or attended to other duties. In all honestly, I like to have a nice jerk off before I start my day. I'm not kidding. Some people like coffee (I do too actually), but I find nothing starts my day off on the right foot like busting a nut.

What Is There To Learn Anyway?

I am certain that if you are reading this work, you have also discovered, with marked curiosity, the jungle gym in your pants. Curiosity is natural and there is nothing wrong with that either. You've probably even jerked off too. You might wonder what else is there to do? Well, let's do a little analogy. Imagine that you are sixteen and you have just passed your driving license exam. Do you think you are ready to go take a race car out on a professional track? Hardly. Just because you have learned to do something marginally correct does not mean that you are ready to turn pro. There are a lot of options out there and a lot of ideas. This book aims to introduce you to many of those ideas. Some you might like and some might not be your thing. That's great. That's what sex is and solo sex is no different. It's a salad bar. If you don't like beets, leave 'em off your salad, but you know they're there is you want to give them a go. This book is your auto erotic salad bar and I'd be very surprised indeed if you did not find something new, useful or interesting in it's pages.

A Quick Note

This book is addressed as a "general adult" title. It is designed as a frank discussion for men of all age about masturbation and it's place in your life. No one will be excluded or left out. However, since the audience can be any adult, I have to assume a tone that is "general". What this means is that I will be talking to men at every point along the sexual road from people who have never even touched their own cock, to people who have not had sexual intercourse, to men who have an orgy with a six pack of broads every Thursday.

What I must ask from you, the reader, is a bit of patience. Please bear with me, and if the narrative is dwelling on a subject with which you are quite familiar, you have my permission to skip ahead. No one will fail this course by skipping ahead. I can promise you that much.

The Benefits Of Masturbation

Practice Makes Perfect

Star athletes and world record holders got there because they are good at what they do and they practiced to get good at their sport. To be good at something, you have to work at it. Why would sex be any different? If you want to be a good lover, you are going to need to learn how your body works, where your pleasure buttons are and how to control yourself. If you don't want to go through life being a two minute man or a two pump chump, you better pencil in some self exploration and masturbation time. Yes, I'm serious. To be a good lover with a partner, man or woman, you need to be a good lover on your own first. I can promise you that no one ever told you that in school.

Why is this the case? It's all about control. Every man, at some point in his life has worried about being too quick. Now I will be the first to tell you that "quick" is sometimes good and sometimes inevitable. It is good when you and your lover are fucking in the public bathroom of a sports arena or concert and need to finish before someone notices. It is also inevitable your first time. You can pull your pork until doomsday, you will not last long your first time. It is just impossible. The frank reality is that you are just too excited at actually getting to use your cock and biology just takes over.

However, the rest of the time, I am pretty sure that you would like some control over your orgasm and how long sex lasts. Ideally, this is because you will have a deep appreciation for the special connection that exists between two people, but in practical terms as well, I am sure you do not look forward to seeing persistent disappointment in the eyes of your lover(s).

Consistent masturbation will allow you to develop the control you need to correct this problem. Most men outgrow this little problem and this is definitely how you do it. Additionally, masturbation will give you an understanding of your orgasm. You will learn when you are getting close to cumming and when to slow down. We will talk more about this more when we delve into technique.

Masturbation Is 100% Safe Sex

Nobody fancies the idea of getting herpes from a hooker or knocking up their girlfriend unexpectedly. These are just a few of the potholes that lie on the road of sex. In all seriousness, sex and its repercussions are very adult indeed. There are problems that can occur that have lasting impact on the life or lives of the participants. I am not trying to scare you. Sex is a wonderful part of a healthy adult life. However, like everything, there is a time and a place and a right and a wrong way to do it.

Frankly, sometimes, sex with a partner is just not a good idea or not an option. If you are young, rushing into sex might seem like a good idea, but sometimes its not. A lot of the time, you are so eager to "get some" you really don't care about who you get it from. When I was growing up, I knew a guy who lost his virginity to a hooker. Not a good idea. Now, to my knowledge, he did not get some horrible STD or knock her up, but he missed out an a special experience. He cheapened it.

Maybe for one reason or another, sex is not right for you at this point in your life. A friend of mine recently went through a painful divorce. Just because he was getting divorced didn't put his sexual desires on hold. However, given his emotional state and the fact his life was in tatters, a relationship was out of the question. That only left casual sex, professional sex (again, hookers) or whacking it. Well, whacking it was the best option. He joked once over beer that he did so around the clock. However, again, it was the best option and it got him through.

Masturbation will never result in a sore that you need to discuss with your doctor or in a baby that needs to get changed every 20 minutes. You can count on that.

Mood Benefits

Masturbation has great mood benefits. When we orgasm, all kinds of healthy chemicals that promote a sense of well being and happiness are released. These chemicals, called endorphins, are the same chemicals that are produced in the brain when people use drugs. Now they are not released in the same quantity, and I want to make sure that you understand that I do not mean masturbating is the same as drug use. Quite the opposite is true!

Masturbation, like drug use, promotes a sense of happiness and well being, however, it does so through a healthy, natural method. Masturbation good, drug use bad.

Sexual release is an important part of your overall sexual health and, if a partner is not available, masturbation is a great option. Honestly, I use it as a calming technique. Think of it as messy, fun meditation. You come home from a rough day, rub one out, and suddenly everything looks a little sunnier. No drugs involved, just a towel. Try it and tell me I'm wrong. Go on. I dare you.

Fun

Let's not kid ourselves, masturbation is fun. Yes, it is not as fun as real sex, but cake is always pretty good, even when it's kinda crappy. This is another major reason that men masturbate. Sometimes it's two in the morning, you're bored and you have to do something. Well, jerking off is a good way to kill the time. You'll have a blast, even though you're alone.

Safe Exploration

Unfortunately, our bodies don't come with an instruction manual and they really should. Things are complicated. Nobody would blame you for being confused. Well, masturbation can help there too. From empirical evidence, most men achieve orgasm for the first time simply by accident. They start rubbing, it feels good and before they know it, they have a mess on their hands. Well, great discoveries are often accidents. Just look at the Americas and penicillin.

However, once this accidental discovery is made, curiosity sets in that really doesn't ever stop. You want to know what you can do with this thing between your legs and what are the limits. So you set of on a natural path of discovery. This is great. When you get a chance to have sex, you will know how your body works and what to do with all those pieces.

Great For Relieving Sexual Tension & Frustration

Sexual tension and frustration can be a real pain in the ass. Imagine that you and your girlfriend broke up a couple of months ago. You haven't gotten laid in 8 weeks. That sucks and things are getting a little backed up as they are apt to do. No one would blame you for feeling tense and frustrated on the sexual scene.

However, that cute girl that runs the coffee stand gave you her number and you two are supposed to go out on a date on Saturday. Great! But, there is one big problem. Just the idea of making love to this woman is driving you nuts. You can't go out like this. You're a volcano about to explode! Your desperation and frustration will be obvious and will actually drive this woman away. You've got to be composed and cool for your date. Women love that. How do you do this?

Don't worry. Masturbation, your trusty friend, has you covered. All you need to do is jerk off a couple of times during the day before you go out. You'll be a bit tapped out and you'll be the calm, cool self that she was attracted to. Think of it like drugging a tiger before you go make it jump through hoops at a magic show. A drugged tiger makes the crowd happy and gets lots of applause. The effect will wear off, but by then, she will be into you and you will be well on your way back to lots of sex with a partner. Thanks masturbation!

Sometimes A Relationship Just Isn't An Option

If you're like me, when you were growing up, you imagined that your life was going to be one big stroll through the garden. Everything was going to work out and you would never have any problems, especially on the relationship front. Then, one ugly day, reality set in. The truth of the matter is that being an adult man, means that sometimes you can be single, even when you don't want to be.

Sometimes a relationship is just not an option. Maybe you're going through a divorce (50% of us will), maybe you work on an oil rig in the ocean, maybe your gay in a small rural ranch town, maybe you're in a monastery, the military, maybe jail. The list is long and there are plenty more reasons that a relationship just isn't an option for you.

There is nothing wrong with this. It's just an ugly fact that we need to get comfortable on our own from time to time. But don't worry, your right hand (or even lefty) will always be there for you. They go where you go and will never break up with you or cheat on you. Plus, your hand is always down to fuck.

The Three Rules To Masturbating Like A Gentleman

We live in a society. As a result, we need to be considerate of others. In this section, I want to go over a few basic rules that will make your masturbation more fun for you and tolerable to those around you.

Making Sure You're Not Interrupted

Just about every man has one. The story where someone, usually a mother or wife depending on their age, walks in on them or almost walked in on them when they were rubbing one out. Now, you should never hide masturbation from your partner, but that is not the point of this blurb.

The point is this. Man came out of the trees and involved into the smartest and most technically advanced creatures to ever walk the face of this planet. Why, with all out abilities, we still get caught with our underwear around our ankles while we are beating our meat is beyond me. This should never happen. Be a man. You have options. Pick somewhere you will not be disturbed (bathroom) and make sure there is a lock on the door. It's that simple. Make an investment now, because seeing the bulging eyes of your mother while you are pumping the bishop is one bucket of ice water. You don't want to experience it. Trust me. That memory never goes away!

Be Careful About Where You Choke Your Chicken

When I was younger, a girlfriend of mine needed a ride to a job interview. I took her, as I am a gentleman, and I waited in the parking lot. Well, it wasn't long before I discovered the adult magazine that I had somehow stashed below my

seat. Honestly, I don't know where it came
from, but some things you just don't question.
Now I love looking at some dirty pictures so I
began to peruse the magazine – again, like a
gentleman.

One thing led to another, and before I knew it, I
was pitching quite the tent. The parking lot
seemed deserted, and I looked around to make
sure no one was around. I was in the clear for a
little self love. I had time to kill and needed to
do something. Well, I whipped it out and
furiously beat it for all of 45 seconds, and I
finished up. I felt pretty good (remember
endorphins).

Then I made a HORRIBLE discovery.
Apparently, I was parked right under one of the
many security cameras. To my horror, it was
pointing right into my car! I had actually
stopped and bopped my bologna right under a
damn security camera.

I was busted. Nothing happened to me that day.
However, for the next five years or so, I waited
for my "candid" camera performance to appear
on some network blooper show. It never did,
but I am sure some security guard had fun

telling his friends about the jackass at work that day.

I tell you this story, my story, as a way to illustrate a point. Be careful about where you choke your chicken. When you are younger, everywhere seems like a good place. However, they're not. Keep it private and behind closed doors. You may be jerking off, but you need to jerk off like a gentleman.

Cleaning Up After Yourself

The first time I was in a dorm, we had a bit of a problem. A dorm, coed or not, is really just a big building filled with young people living on their own for the first time. Not everyone is getting laid, and everyone is horny all the time. Nothing wrong with that. However, it is not surprising that under the roof of a dorm, there is a lot of masturbation happening. Well, there is another problem. You almost always have a roommate and, as good a friends as you may be, you don't want to watch each other jerk off. So you use the showers.

Well, in this dorm, some ass was not cleaning up after himself. He would just spunk on the wall or floor of the shower and leave it. One, this is not OK. Two, let that be a lesson to take some shower shoes with you when you live in a dorm. Stepping in something that looks a lot like semen on the floor of a public shower is not fun for anyone.

Again, as a gentleman masturbator, you have responsibilities. Nothing is more important than cleaning up after yourself. Make it happen every time.

Basic Masturbation Techniques

In this section, we are going to go through the "basics" that a man needs to know to thoroughly enjoy masturbation. These techniques are intended for frequent use.

Don't Forget Foreplay

Men really just are not good at foreplay. When we get the idea of sex in our brain, we always seem to assume that our bodies are ready (the bodies of our lovers too). Well, the truth of the matter is a bit different. Your car needs a minute to warm up to work optimally and your cock and balls are no different.

Don't just start pulling on your limp dick and expect everything to be A-OK. Instead, get into the practice of allowing yourself a little time to warm up. Watch a little adult video material. Rub some warming oil on your package and give it a little massage. You get the idea.

However, if you do this, you will accomplish two things that will make your sex life better. The first is that you will learn to relax a little and enjoy your masturbation more. Yep, more. The second is that you will teach yourself (mind and body) to wait a little in terms of sex. This is a great skill to have and is one that your many future lovers will appreciate. A man who can wait a little to get laid will have more sex, better sex, and sex more often in the future. Both the ladies and the gents will appreciate a man who takes his time to do it right. Start now!

The Standard Technique

In the standard masturbation technique, a man lies down on a bed. This technique can also be applied in the seated position, although I prefer lying down. There is a certain freedom in lying down and I find that you can close your eyes and enjoy more.

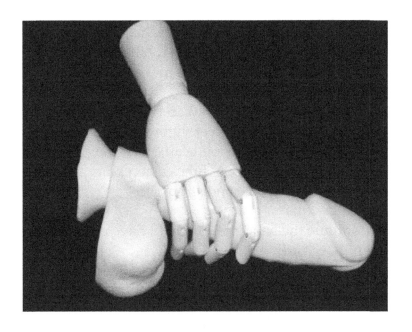

With your dominant hand, grasp your erect cock and apply some lube. Wrap your fingers around the shaft of the penis, and begin a gentle up and down motion along the shaft. With this technique, you are essentially creating a fake vagina (or anus if you like) with your hand. You are then allowing the "fake" to fuck your cock.

Pressure is definitely something you want to play with here. You can go loose if you want to tease yourself, or you can squeeze very tightly. I would, as with all of these basic techniques, encourage you to play with the grip. Start loose and then go tight or vice versa. You can also vary it throughout the act to make it a lot of fun.

If you are circumcised, be careful around the helmet of the penis. Over vigorous masturbation at this point can cause chaffing. Also, continue to apply lube as necessary. You want to keep it nice and slippery.

Continue the hand motion that I have described until orgasm.

Alternating Hands

Alternating hands is a lot of fun with masturbation and can add variety, the spice of life, to the act.

Too often, I find that men use the same technique to jerk off all the time. This can be a big problem. It trains your cock and your mind to expect that kind of stimulation each and every time. This is fine if you are serving a 25 year prison term with limited social possibilities. However, if you are sexually active, you cannot expect real sex to offer this kind of stimulation. This can result in men being able to orgasm only though masturbation. This in turn is frustrating and will make you miss out on the joys of actual sex.

Throughout this work, I am going to encourage you to spice it up and not to allow this problem to occur for you. Switching hands is just the first step you can take. When you choke your chicken with the left hand and you are a righty, you will experience a different sensation and a different style. It may be hard to cum at first, but you will get there and the extra time it takes to reach orgasm will mean that the orgasm you experience is a stronger, more enjoyable one.

Fucking Your Hand

Fucking your hand is another masturbation technique, and in combination with "The Standard Technique" should form the core of your masturbation repetoire. With this technique, it is not your hand that moves, but your body, as you rhythmically fuck your own hand.

To begin this position, lie on your side on your bed, or somewhere else flat and comfortable. Apply plenty of lube to your hand and then grab hold of your cock in the manner shown in the

picture below. You will notice that the ring
made by your thumb and forefinger are at the
base of your penis. This of course is completely
opposite to "The Standard Technique".

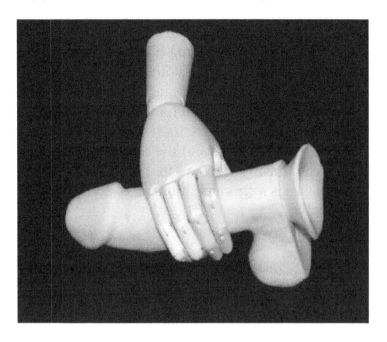

Now, to carry out this position, you will now
move your hips backwards and forwards. This
will move your cock in and out of your hand,
just like it would a vagina (or again, anus). With
this position, you will find the sensation to be
quite different, in a pleasing manner. This is

actually very close to the sensation (physically speaking at least) of actual sexual intercourse.

One thing that you want to consider is laying down a towel for you to lie on. When you cum, it is entirely possible to cum all over the bed with this position. A towel will keep the mess to a bare minimum.

This position has two advantages that you should be aware of. First, it mixes up the sensation and does not make you dependent on one particular type of sensation. Two, it is also a great hip workout. Hip motion and the ability to do that for a while are an essential criteria to being a good lover when the time comes to actually have sex. This position will help you get used to that act and will help to condition the relevant muscles. Plus, it feels really good.

Double Handed Sword

With the double handed sword, it is best to be by lying down on a bed again. Grab hold of your erect cock with your dominant hand. Then, wrap your other hand around the dominant hand. Now, begin to move your hands up and down over your erect penis. As usual play with the tightness to increase your pleasure.

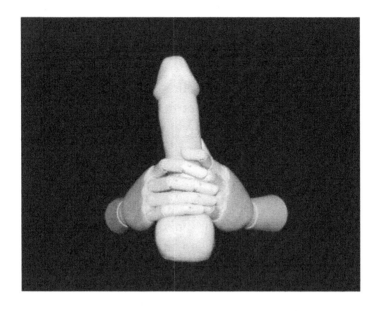

This technique may not seem like to much of a change from the normal routine, but it can have a lot of difference in your fantasy. If you are stroking over the whole of your unit, your forearms will be slapping against your pelvis. This creates an almost identical feeling to someone sitting on your cock. I guarantee if you close your eyes and picture the person of your choice bouncing up and down on your throbbing member, while using this technique, you will have a whole new world of fantasy to

play in and you'll be cumming in no time! No
need to thank me.

Pulling The Taffy

Normal masturbation techniques employ your
hand (up to this point) moving up and down
along the shaft of your cock. However, have you
ever thought of going just one way? That is
what this technique does. Since it eliminates half
of the normal action, it is not unexpected that
this technique takes longer. While it takes
longer, it also heightens the excitement and
pleasure and draws out the fun. It is definitely
worth trying both ways before you make your
final decision.

To start, lie down and romance yourself a bit.
Once you have an erection, lube it up and take
your dominant hand and grasp your penis.
Now, move your hand up the shaft of your
penis. As you do so, as part of the same motion,
begin to grab hold of your penis with your non-
dominant hand and begin to move it up.
Repeat this process back and forth between your
two hands. Your hand will always move up
along your cock and as one finishes the other
begins. Your cock will always be receiving
stimulation, but only in one direction.

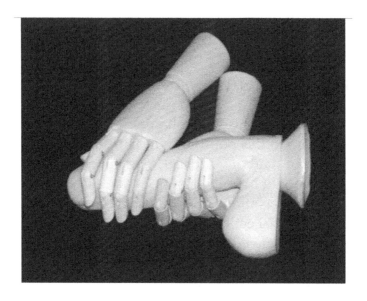

To mix things up, you can reverse everything and only move down your cock towards your balls. This is a great handjob technique and it works just as well on yourself as it does with a partner. While you are doing this, feel free to play with the speed of your hands as much as the tightness of the grip.

Standing Hand Fuck

This technique is a perfect one for the shower, which makes clean up a breeze. If you choose to use it somewhere other than in the shower, make sure that you have a plan for cleanup or you will be spunking all over the place.

To carry out the standing hand fuck, pick a nice place to stand. Grasp your erection in the same manner as shown in the "Fucking Your Hand" section. Add lube and begin to pump into your hand. Since you are standing, you will now have full use of your leg muscles. This maneuver will give you the real sense of bending someone over and fucking them. This is a real treat and will add a bit of dominant spice to your solo sex life.

One bit of advice. When you are cumming, your legs may become a little wobbly. First off, be aware of this and prepare accordingly. Secondly, to brace yourself, you can use your free hand and rest along a wall.

An Introduction To Male Masturbators

Jerking off is all well and good. It is fun to lie on a bed and pump yourself to orgasm over and over, however, sometimes, you long for variety. Meet the masturbator. A masturbator in short, is a sex toy designed for use by men, during masturbation, that offers more pleasure and realism than could be achieved by the hand alone.

There are many kinds of masturbators out there. There are pussy and even anus shaped ones. There are all kinds of varying degrees of tightness and internal pleasure mechanisms. Vibrating and warming pocket pussies are also very common. One of my favorite types of masturbators are silicone rubber in the exact shape of famous porn starlets vaginas. It's as close as you can get to the real thing.

There are also different styles. There are handheld masturbators that are used as a more pleasurable version of a man's hand. With these, he moves them up and down until he cums. There are also fully sized vaginas and even sex dolls that will offer you a chance to really get in there and have some sex.

With masturbators and sex dolls, I will caution you to go to a store and actually do some investigation before you buy something. There are, unfortunately, some poorly made sex toys out there. There is nothing worse than spending $100 for a masturbator, getting all excited about giving it a go, only to find out that it pinches your cock when you use it. It happens and it sucks! If you go to a reputable sex toy supplier, they will have no problem letting you inspect the merchandise before buying it. With sex toys, of course, there is no return and you want to make sure you are getting your money's worth the first time around.

Fucking The Bed

The idea of fucking the bed, or at least the space between the mattress and box spring occurs to many, many men. You are there in your private bedroom, you're horny, and with just a little imagination, you can see how that slit might offer you a very close approximation to real pussy.

Well, in all honesty, you are right. That slit will offer you a chance to simulate a pussy quite well. However, you need to go about it the right way. There are some problems that need to be overcome.

The biggest problems are lubrication and mess. The space between a bed and box spring is neither wet, nor slippery. This means if you fuck it as is, you are going to do nothing more than give your cock some serious friction burns. This is to be avoided.

The best way to handle this is with a plastic bag. A sandwich bag works wonderfully well. Avoid the "locking" types. Take this bag and fill it with the lube of your choice. Not all the way, but liberally apply it to the inside of the bag. For my part, I prefer a water based lube. If you use something like petroleum jelly, you can stain the bed if you're not careful. Nobody wants a mystery stain on their mattress. It is pretty awkward to flip it then.

Now, take the bag that is full of lube and put your cock in it. Then, slip the whole cock/bag assembly into the slit and get comfortable. Make sure your unit isn't being crushed. When you're comfortable start fucking away! It's actually quite enjoyable. If you need more lube, pause and reload the bag as you go.

The bag system works great for cleaning up as well. You fuck the bag and you cum in the bag. No mess in the bed. A condom might be used as a substitution, but in my experience, condoms are likely to break with this kind of activity. They are just not designed for that level of friction. Then, you've go a mess on your hands.

Vibrators

Vibrators are not just for women. They feel great on men too. With vibrators, you have a couple of options. You can get a vibrating masturbator. These are often called "pocket pussies". Essentially, this is a vagina (or anus) shaped masturbator that has a built in, multi-speed, vibrating function. Honestly, I wish I could give these a better recommendation. I really wanted to like these, but I find them to be less than pleasing. You see, a vagina doesn't vibrate. It just makes sex with a vibrating one, even a fake one, less than my cup of tea.

Where vibrators really come into their own is as a small vibrating unit. Bullets are very small vibrators (about 2 inches in length) that offer portable, waterproof, concentrated stimulation. On the tip of your penis, soft or hard, they are guaranteed to get a reaction. I can promise you that.

I strongly recommend that you go get a vibrator and keep it next to your bed. Play with it. Get used to its stimulation. A man who is comfortable with a vibrator and knows how to use one properly will find that their sexual partners come back for more. You will know what you like and how to make your partner feel great at the same time.

To find a vibrator, you can go to your friendly neighborhood adult boutique, or you can shop online. There are plenty or retailers that will be happy to help you find what you are looking for.

There is one place to buy that you may have overlooked however. This is your friendly neighborhood, big box, health section. Many of these stores, in the "massager area" sell very powerful, intense and pleasurable vibrators. They plug into the wall and they may call them "back massagers" but they vibrate really well and you will never need to look for batteries. Nothing worse than running out of batteries for your vibrator whether you are alone or with a partner. These babies only stop when they shut off the electricity.

Anal Play

I am not the biggest fan of anal play for personal reasons, but I am also all about empowerment. Many people are curious about working their anus into their masturbation routine and enjoy it when they do. Let me set the record straight right here and say that this is OK. There are a lot of nerve endings in the anus that make stimulation in that area, especially in concert with jerking off a lot of fun. A vibrator down there while you are really choking your chicken can be quite a treat indeed.

If you do choose to do some anal play, start in the shower. This makes it really easy to clean up if you make a mess.

Instant Noodle Masturbator

When you're young and curious you will try anything once. Having sex with an instant noodle cup was one of those things for me. Honestly, it makes a pretty good homemade masturbator and they cost even less than a watermelon. Here is how you can make one.

- Make a normal instant noodle cup. Follow the instructions on the package.
- Drain the hot water leaving only noodles in the cup.
- Tape up the top of the noodle cup and cut a penis sized hole in it.

- **Wait until the noodles cool to desired temp. Insert your finger to make sure that the noodles have cooled to a safe temperature. Do not move to step 5 until you are certain the noodles have cooled.**
- Masturbate using your cup of noodle masturbation toy. Using it as a replacement for your hand in "The Standing Hand Fuck" works great.
- If the noodles get cold, just lightly microwave them. Follow step 4 before continuing.

If for some reason, you cannot or will not buy a masturbation toy, consider this option for making one at home. No one looks at a guy with a case of instant noodles funny. Believe me, I stood in line with them plenty of times.

Watermelons

You might be laughing right now, but the truth is that fucking a watermelon is actually a lot of fun. I am not saying that it is more desirable than actually having sex, but if your alone, bored and have a watermelon, I have something for you to try.

You're reading this so I will assume that you are a smart guy, but I will give you a quick run down on how to turn a watermelon into a home made fuck toy. Here goes:

- Cut a circular hole in the rind of the watermelon using a kitchen knife. You are just cutting a hole in the skin. You are not carving out something to fuck just yet.
- Remove the circular piece of rind.
- Take a long thin knife and carve out a passage way into the watermelon.
- Have fun. Lots of fun.

When I was younger, this was a popular topic of discussion, and being a curious young man, I gave it a try. People always talked about microwaving the melon beforehand. Think of it as watermelon foreplay. This was never my thing. A watermelon warming in the summer sun was always just right. Cold wasn't fun either so avoid a watermelon from the fridge, although, you can try it if you like. If you do, don't be surprised if you lose your erection.

Slow Masturbation

Slow masturbation is not so much a technique in and of itself, but is more of an "add on" that you can pair up with any of the techniques so far mentioned in this book.

With slow masturbation, you draw out the time it takes you to reach orgasm and in the process heighten and intensify the resulting orgasm. The approach is simple. Stroke very slowly for a while, then quickly stroke for a short amount of time. As a rule, start with 30 slow strokes and 15 fast. Repeat as desired until orgasm is reached.

This practice will really build your orgasm. I guarantee it will be a stronger, more powerful one when it does happen. The wait is really worth it.

Taking It To The Brink – Building Control

I alluded, in the introduction, to how masturbation can build your control and make you a better lover. Now, I will get into the details of how that works and how you can make it happen.

When you are jerking off, the muscles in your penis tighten and eventually go into a spasm of orgasm that results in ejaculation. This doesn't just happen. It is a gradual build that a man can feel. The first step in learning to control when your orgasm happens and how long you can have sex for, begins with identification. You need to identify the feelings in your penis as you build towards orgasm.

For every man, there is a "point of no return". After you have orgasmed a few times in your life, you will be familiar with this point. What you are aiming to do is approach that point of no return, get as close to it as possible, and then slow down. When you slow down, the orgasm will retreat away (in most cases) while your cock remains hard. This will allow you to continue masturbating (or fucking if you are with a partner) and enjoying yourself. This can, in theory, be done many times allowing you to prolong your lovemaking beyond the reach of men who have not trained in this way. No more "quick draw" for you.

I said that in "most cases" your orgasm will retreat. This is true, but what happens when it doesn't? Well, two things can happen. The first and most obvious event that can happen is that you go ahead and cum. If this happens, you got to close to the "point of no return" and overshot the mark. Not a big deal. Next time, slow it down a little sooner. Learn from the mistake and enjoy the post orgasm high that you get.

However, there is another possibility. Men who have a lengthier history of sexual activity will be aware of this, but those without might not be. You can "miss" all together. When your cock is being stimulated (either by you or a partner) and you are building towards orgasm, there is a certain window of opportunity for you to cum. Sometimes, if you change up the stimulation during that period (like, for example, right before the "point of no return") things just go wrong and you don't orgasm no matter what happens. This can happen easily and most likely will at some point in your life. Your cock goes limp and you're done for a bit. If this happens, don't panic! Everything is OK. Think of orgasms as a bus. If you miss one, try again in 15 minutes. Everything will have reset by then.

Hopefully, by applying the technique that I have just described, you will build your control and become a better, more pleasing lover. Additionally, you will be able to have sex for longer periods of time. Men who can control their orgasm and can extend lovemaking beyond the length of a commercial break get laid much more often. I can assure you of that!

Jerking Off With A Partner

Masturbation is not necessarily a solo activity. If no one has ever told you that, now you know. Masturbation is simply the act of pleasuring yourself. No one ever said you had to be alone in the room to do it.

If you haven't ever jerked off with your partner you should definitely consider exploring it, once you have talked to them. There is a lot to be gained.

First of all, it is really hot. You are watching them and they are watching you and the two of you are feeding off each other's excitement and arousal. This is one of those times when your control training will cum in handy. A normal man, the first time they get to watch their partner's auto erotic activities will bust a nut in no time. Not you! You can handle it and know when to slow down to keep the party going.

Secondly, there is a lot that a couple can learn by engaging in this activity. The person who best knows how to pleasure someone is themselves. They know their body best and they know best how they like to be touched. Watching them play with themselves and observing how it is done is as close as you will ever get to being in their head.

The same goes for you. If you want your partner to know how to touch you and to give you the maximum amount of sexual pleasure, it would be foolish to assume that they know how to do it perfectly based on instinct. You have to show them and teach them. Everyone is different and we all enjoy different sensations. Offer your lover a window into your soul by permitting them to watch you masturbate.

Thirdly, masturbating with your partner is a way to build trust and intimacy, through a sexual act that is deeply personal, yet at the same time is completely disease free with no risk of pregnancy. If for one reason or another, you cannot engage in traditional sexual activity, this achieves many of the same results without any of the potential problems of other sexual acts. Plus, as a couple, you can still bathe in the afterglow.

If you are in a relationship, and this activity has never been discussed, you should consider it. It is a lot of fun and, like I said, there is a lot to learn. Also, it is great foreplay if you do wish to engage in actual sex. Everyone will be all warmed up and ready to go for some hot, wild sex. Trust me.

Use Your Imagination From Time To Time

It makes me feel old to say this, but when I was growing up, we did not have porn like there is today. We would buy crumpled, crusty magazines stolen from under dad's beds. Maybe someone would get lucky from time to time and score a VHS. Not a DVD, but a VHS. From time to time, we would be out of luck and we would have to use our imaginations.

This is not the case today. Streaming internet porn is available 24 hours a day, every day and can be found by simply clicking a button. No fees. Free and abundant porn for everyone. I would be a liar if I told you I wasn't a fan and hadn't used it before. I have. But there is a danger in the constantly available internet porn that you should be aware of.

Our brains our our biggest sexual organs. Yes, our brains. Compared to what is happening in your brain, your cock matters very little. When our brains become accustomed to only being fed a steady stream of raunchy, obscene, off the hook jerk porn, it can become desensitized to regular sex. Think about it. If all you watch every time you jerk off is interracial gang bang S&M porn, making love to your girlfriend (and thus having a healthy, normal adult relationship) might not be enough.

It's OK to watch some wild porn now and again on the internet. However, do yourself a favor. Lie back, close your eyes and just use your mind from time to time. Build your imagination and develop your own sexual fantasies rather than having them spoon fed to you. Have fun and see where it goes. You will be making yourself a better, more creative lover at the same time you are exploring and understanding your own sexuality.

Slippery When Wet

In a work of this kind, I have found that people are always eager to get to the "good stuff". When the subject is masturbation, they are eager to know how to spank their monkey. That is why the "techniques" section was placed above the "lubrication" section. It is best to give the people what they want. However, there is nothing more important to enjoyable masturbation than lubrication. As such, this section, which is playing second fiddle, is actually as important, if not more so than techniques. Without proper lubrication all the above listed techniques will do is chafe your throbbing cock and leave you unsatisfied.

The Importance & Fun Of Lube

A penis is a battering ram. When used according to design, the penis is shoved into a self lubricating vagina and is pumped up and down. Now this is nothing against anyone who want to place their cock into anything other than a vagina. I have, and will do again and let me tell you all of the options out there are a lot of fun for consenting adults. It is just that we are not using the penis as it was intended.

That's where lube comes in. The penis is intended to be surrounded with lubrication to work properly and enjoyably. Thanks to both nature and modern science, we have a lot of options to choose from. We are going to go through all the options that are available to you. It is also important that a man understand lube and lubrication from their partners point of view as well.

Whether it is an ass or a pussy you wish to shove your hard, eager cock into, it needs to be lubed. In the case of a pussy, some foreplay may do the trick, but it may not. In that case, you will need some of the information here. In the case of anal sex, everything that you learn here might be helpful to you in the future. A man that understands lube and knows how to keep their partner comfortably lubricated will go far in the way of finding eager partners.

Spit – Always Handy

Spit really is the best natural lubricant you can find. Yes, saliva. Drooling all over something, be it a pussy, a cock or your hand is one of the best ways that you can quickly and conveniently make it slippery. If you don't believe me, lick your fingers thoroughly and rub them together. You will find that there is quite a bit less friction than there was before.

Saliva makes lubricated masturbation a dream. Grab your hard cock and spit on it a bunch. Slowly rub your hand up and down the shaft as you spread out the spit and cover the whole of the shaft and before you know it you are ready to go. Jerk away! Now the spit will not last forever. Depending on the length and the duration of the masturbation session, you may need to re-wet things. Don't worry. Just spit on it again and you're good to go.

Water Based Lube

For those who suffer from permanent cottonmouth or for those who find the idea of spitting all over their cock to be a little odd, there is water based lube.

Water based lube is sold under a host of brand names and is often sold as a personal lubricant. It is great for sex in that it does not break down condoms and it works for inserting tampons as well. However, for our purposes, it is great for jerking off. It is slipperier than saliva and really gets things gliding along. Don't go nuts when you first apply it or you will waste it.

Water based lubrication is also good in that it is water based. That means it cleans up really easily. Wipe it off with a towel and run it through the washing machine and everything is as good as new. It will just wash away.

To find water based lube look in the pharmacy section of any department store. It is usually sold next to the condoms. If you are embarrassed about buying it (you shouldn't be, everyone jerks off) go through the self check out aisle. No one asks questions there and it is just lube. Not like you're buying cigarettes.

Lotions

Lotion is good for two reasons. First off, for those afraid of buying lube, nobody looks twice when you buy some lotion. Secondly, lotion is found all over the place. This means that when you wish to spontaneously rub one out, lotion is usually close at hand to help you take care of business.

Not just any lotion will do. You want hypoallergenic, scent free lotion. Scents that are added to lotions use chemicals (usually alcohols). This means that you could go pull your pork with a lovely lavender scented lotion only to find your cock covered in a rash a little bit later. The heat and sweat in your undercarriage only help to make this more likely. To find a unscented lotion, just read the bottles. Lotions that are unscented and are hypoallergenic will make no secret about it. That is their big selling point and it should be printed right on the front.

Also, for those of you that have a partner, keeping a bottle of lotion next to the bed can be dual purposed. It is great for rubbing one out when you are home alone. However, it is also great for giving foot rubs when you get company. A man who rubs the feet of his partner will be pulling his pork a lot less. One way or the other, the lotion is handy to have.

Exfoliating Cream

Exfoliating creams are creams with small amounts of abrasives added to them. The abrasives are used to scrub skin smooth. Well, sometime back I wanted to make sure that the skin on my penis was kissably smooth. Well, I'll be damned if I didn't discover how much fun it was to exfoliate your penis skin in the shower. The lotion made a nice lube and I just kept exfoliating until I was finished. It was great and I would (and have) done it many times since.

Warming Lubes

Warming lubes are a newer product on the market but they are a lot of fun to use when you are choking your chicken. Cold lube takes away from the magic of jerking off and serves to remind you that you are alone. With warming lube, we as a society, have taken one more step towards totally "real" jerking off.

Personally, I like these products, I can close my eyes, do the "double handed sword" with some warming lube and easily imagine some buxom woman with her warm pussy bouncing up and down on my cock. Warming lubes are also great for use in a masturbator, again for added realism. To find warming lubes, all you need to do is go to your local grocery store. Again, they are sold in the same areas as condoms. Adult boutiques will have a larger selection but, will find plenty to get you started and experimenting here.

Cloth "Lube"

Pubic hair is not just there for show. It serves a very real purpose. It acts as a lubricant during sex. Now before you go and call me crazy, I want you to try something. Push down hard on the hair on your head with the palm of your hand (you might be reading this in public and I can't have you shoving your hand in your pants) now move it around. What happens? It glides. Now put the palms of your hands together and try to do the same thing. The palms lock up thanks to our old friend "friction". The reason that didn't happen on your head was hair. Your pubic hair does the same thing and allows your nether regions to mix with another persons without chaffing. Mother Nature is pretty cool.

Well, you can use this same line of thinking if you find yourself in a pinch and don't have any lube handy and you don't want to spit on your cock. Use a soft cloth. Wrapping your cock in, say a soft cotton T-shirt, will prevent friction and allow you to jerk off with ease. Towels work pretty well too. Start with a light grip to make sure everything is sliding along and then tighten it.

Going Dry

Some people like to drink vodka straight. Most don't, but some people enjoy it. The same can be said for choking your chicken without any type of lube. I call it "going dry".

There is nothing wrong with this activity, and in fact, it offers a unique and enjoyable form of stimulation. However, you need to be a little careful. Avoid getting it wet. Water only adds to friction and can chafe. If you're going to go dry, it needs to go dry.

One consideration that you should be made aware of is that if you go dry, it can serve to desensitize your penis a bit. This can mean it takes you longer to orgasm in general. However, like so many things that may be considered "bad" for us, it is fun in moderation.

Cleaning Up Can Be Hard To Do

One of the biggest problems with masturbation, at least for us men, is the mess afterward. It can be a bit of a hassle. If you want to go jerk off in the public bathroom at work on a little "break" you need to think about cleanup. The same can be said in the shower, in the bed, etc. However, the reality is that cleanup shouldn't be such a problem. There are a few techniques that I will teach you that will make cleanup a breeze, and it will help you to keep your masturbation habits as private as you would like them to be. Remember, cleaning up after yourself is one of the three rules of jerking off like a gentleman.

Toilet Paper & Paper Towels – The first instinct of most men. Avoid it if you can. It is rough, causes chaffing and can stick on the end of your cock. Not fun at all.

Bath Towels – Bath towels are one of the best options out there. They are absorbent, soft and are usually a color designed to hide stains. Perfect! Throw them in a hamper with other towels and no one needs to know the dirty secret. Of course, is you are on your own and doing your own laundry (hopefully you are) keeping one by the bed for when the mood strikes is a good idea too. Nothing worse than having to pause while you find a towel.

The Shower - The shower is great because it makes clean up unnecessary. Just spunk all you want and you're good to go. Make sure you hose off the wall and get everything. There are precious few people indeed that will not mind stepping into a glob of your cold sperm from when you took a shower last night. Remember, show some courtesy.

Socks Are A Cock's Best Friend – One time, I went to go pick up a friend for a night out on the town. His roommate let me in and told me he was back in his room. We were close so I went and knocked. No answer. Well I opened the door (there is a life lesson in here) and found my friend passed out drunk with a sock around his erection. He had a death grip on the sock too! Well, we all had a good laugh at his expense and still do to this day. However, there is something to this beyond a lesson in knocking.

Socks really are great for clean up purposes. Your cock fits right in them. If you're like most men, you've got them lying around and with a sock you don't need to worry about lube. It's just natural to use them for jerking off. I made fun of my friend, but have used his technique several times since. Put it on your to do list too.

Condoms – Condoms are another clean up solution that seems so obvious but is often overlooked. You've probably got some in the house. They're already pre-lubed and they have that nice reservoir tip on the end. Perfect for solo, no mess, whacking it. Easy.

However, you need to be careful with condoms. Even if you live by yourself. What if your girlfriend comes over and looks in the bathroom waste basket and sees a condom. It wasn't from her. Now you have some explaining to do and the excuse that you were only using it to jerk off will only go so far.

The Toilet – When I'm on the toilet, I am not usually there to jerk off, but, I want to be fair to my readers. As such, I am including this bullet point in our discussion. If you like the sound of this, by all means go for it.

When you're sitting on the toilet, you can very easily direct your penis so you just cum right in the toilet. This is especially true of the elongated oval bowl designs. This works especially well if you need a jerk break at work. No evidence to leave behind and, provided you are eager enough, you can even pull this one (no pun intended) off in a stall.

Wet Naps – Where toilet paper falls short, wet naps go the distance. Wet naps are designed for serious clean up of delicate tissues. Also, since they are moistened (and even treated with aloe) they don't stick.   Pocket a few extra the next time you are eating BBQ, or if you find some on the back of the toilet the next time you are rubbing one out, feel free to use them. They have the seal of approval.

Dirty Laundry – In the same vein as socks, dirty laundry is also great for taking care of business. If you live like I did when I was single, there is probably dirty clothes on the floor in front of you while you read this. Well, it's going in the laundry anyway and detergent has no problem getting out cum stains, so...why not? For me, I like the cotton T-shirts the best. I am talking about those undershirt ones. They are soft and absorbent and will do the trick just fine.

Conclusion

Well, there it is. That is what I have for you at this point. Hopefully, you have learned some fun new techniques that you can go out and try. Maybe I have described something that piqued your interest of has allowed you to look at masturbating in a fun new light. That was my goal. It is my sincere hope that you have enjoyed this work and found reading it as much fun as I have found writing it. Good luck and happy chicken choking!

Made in the USA
Monee, IL
07 October 2023

44123424R10038